METHYLENE BLUE

Unleashing the Healing Power, Medical and Industrial Applications of the Amazingly Versatile Wonder Dye

By

Jeanne B. Meyer

Copyright @2023

TABLE OF CONTENT

Methylene blue is a compound known for its impressive versatility and extensive range of applications. Methylene blue has demonstrated its effectiveness and versatility across various applications, including medical diagnostics, treatments, scientific research, and industrial processes. This book delves into the world of a remarkable substance, examining its various uses in areas such as diagnostic staining, treatment of methemoglobinemia, neuroprotective effects, potential benefits, and recent advancements in its application. This comprehensive guide explores the various applications of methylene blue and its significant impact across industries such as medicine, photography, and wastewater treatment.

Methylene blue's medical applications and remarkable potential include, but are not limited to:

Malaria: Malaria has been discovered to be treatable with methylene blue.

Memory decline: Even outside of dementia, the antioxidant activity of methylene blue may help prevent age-related injury.

Lyme disease: Researchers examined medications that eliminate the Lyme disease-causing bacteria. Methylene blue was effective at eradicating antibiotic-resistant bacteria in the laboratory.

Cancer: It has been used particularly to detect gastrointestinal cancers, overactive parathyroid glands, and lymph node cancer.

Alzheimer's disease: Researchers are investigating the potential of methylene to reduce memory loss in Alzheimer's dementia patients.

Come along with us as we explore the mysteries and possibilities of this intriguing and lifesaving compound.

CHAPTER ONE

Introduction to Methylene Blue

Methylene Blue is classified as a synthetic compound and is a member of the thiazine dye family. The substance is notable for its deep blue hue and has found extensive use across multiple industries owing to its wide range of properties and applications. Methylene blue is composed of a tricyclic phenothiazine ring system that includes a central nitrogen atom, as observed in its chemical structure. The distinctive color of methylene blue is attributed to its structure, which enables it to interact with various molecules. As a result, methylene blue finds utility in a wide range of processes.

Methylene Blue has a significant historical background as it was initially synthesized during the 19th century. The technology has been widely utilized in various fields including medicine, biology, chemistry, and industry. The versatility of this substance can be attributed to its distinct properties, such as its capability to function as a redox indicator, an electron carrier, and an antimicrobial agent.

Methylene blue has been widely used in the field of medicine for a range of purposes. The utilization of this substance as a diagnostic dye has proven to be beneficial in enhancing the visualization of tissues and biological specimens in various medical procedures, including histology and surgical mapping. Methylene blue is commonly used as a treatment for methemoglobinemia, which is a medical condition that causes a decrease in the blood's ability to carry oxygen. In addition, recent studies have investigated the potential neuroprotective effects of [subject] and its application in photodynamic therapy for specific types of cancer.

In addition to its use in medicine, methylene blue has various applications in other fields. In laboratory settings, it is commonly employed as a staining agent and in a variety of biochemical assays. The utilization of this substance has been observed in various industrial processes, including the dyeing of textiles, as well as its application in photography and artistic endeavors. In addition, it is worth noting that methylene blue possesses antimicrobial properties and has been utilized in various applications such as water treatment and environmental purposes.

It is crucial to acknowledge that methylene blue, despite its many advantages and uses, also carries potential side effects and factors to consider. It is important to adhere to proper handling, storage, and usage guidelines in order to prioritize safety and prevent any potential negative consequences. Methylene blue demonstrates versatility and has made substantial contributions across multiple fields. The unique properties and applications of this subject are currently being investigated, leading to ongoing research and innovation.

Chemical Properties and Structure of Methylene Blue

Methylene Blue is a synthetic compound that possesses a complex chemical structure and exhibits distinct properties, which play a significant role in its diverse range of applications. Let us examine the chemical properties and structure of it.

Methylene Blue is classified as a member of the thiazine dye family and possesses a core structure consisting of a tricyclic phenothiazine ring system. The compound is composed of three benzene rings (A, B, and C rings) that are fused together, with nitrogen atoms located at positions 3 and 7. The positive charge of the compound is attributed to the central nitrogen atom, which is commonly referred to as the N^+ ion.

The molecular formula of Methylene Blue, $C_{16}H_{18}ClN_3S$, indicates the presence of carbon, hydrogen, chlorine, nitrogen, and sulfur atoms in its composition. The molecular weight of the substance is approximately 319.85 g/mol.

The spectral properties of Methylene Blue are characterized by its ability to absorb and reflect specific wavelengths of light, resulting in a deep blue color. The material exhibits a notable absorption peak within the visible light spectrum, specifically in the range of 660-665 nm. This characteristic contributes to its vibrant blue coloration. The compound's absorption and reflection properties contribute to its utility in staining and visualizing biological specimens across a range of applications.

The solubility and stability of Methylene Blue are important factors to consider. It is known to be water-soluble, meaning it can easily dissolve in aqueous solutions. The solubility of the substance enables convenient preparation of solutions with specific concentrations, catering to various applications. The compound exhibits stability under typical conditions; however, it may undergo degradation when exposed to light and air. Proper storage in opaque containers and protection from excessive light exposure are crucial factors in maintaining the stability of the substance.

Methylene Blue exhibits reversible redox reactions as a significant property. The compound has the ability to both accept and donate electrons, which gives it valuable properties as a redox indicator and electron carrier in a range of chemical and biological processes. The compound has the ability to exist in two different forms: oxidized (Methylene Blue) and reduced (Leucomethylene Blue). This property allows it to actively participate in electron transfer reactions.

The chemical properties and distinct structure of Methylene Blue play a significant role in its wide array of applications. These include its utilization as a diagnostic dye, antimicrobial agent, and electron carrier in redox reactions. Gaining knowledge about the chemical properties of a substance enhances our understanding of its usefulness and lays the groundwork for investigating its diverse applications across various disciplines.

CHAPTER TWO

Medical and Clinical Applications

The medical and clinical applications of methylene blue are diverse and significant. Methylene blue is a versatile dye that has been used in various medical procedures and treatments. It has been employed as a diagnostic tool, particularly in urology, to identify and visualize abnormalities

The unique properties and versatile nature of Methylene Blue have led to its significant medical and clinical applications across various fields. Let's examine some of the noteworthy applications of it.

Methylene Blue is commonly utilized as a diagnostic stain in medical and laboratory environments. The application of this substance can be either topical or through injection. Its purpose is to stain tissues, which enhances the ability to visualize and distinguish structures during various procedures, including histology, cytology, and surgical mapping.

The treatment of methemoglobinemia involves addressing the abnormal increase in methemoglobin, which is a type of hemoglobin that is unable to effectively transport oxygen. Methylene Blue functions as a reducing agent, enabling the conversion of methemoglobin into functional hemoglobin. This process effectively restores the capacity of hemoglobin to carry oxygen. In emergency situations, methemoglobinemia is treated by administering it intravenously.

Methylene Blue exhibits antimicrobial properties, effectively targeting various bacteria, viruses, and fungi. The ability to inhibit microbial growth is achieved through the disruption of their metabolic processes and the damage inflicted on their cell membranes. In clinical practice, the topical application of certain medications may be utilized as a treatment for specific skin infections. Additionally, it can be used in conjunction with other therapies to help manage microbial conditions.

According to research, Methylene Blue has been found to potentially possess neuroprotective properties. The potential benefits of this substance include its ability to reduce oxidative stress, alleviate neuroinflammation, and improve mitochondrial function. These effects could have positive implications for individuals with neurological conditions like Alzheimer's disease and Parkinson's disease. Nevertheless, additional research is currently being conducted to determine the efficacy of this treatment in these specific domains.

Photodynamic Therapy (PDT) is a treatment method that utilizes Methylene Blue. This therapy involves using light to activate a photosensitive compound, which then generates reactive oxygen species. These reactive oxygen species are responsible for destroying specific cells, such as cancer cells. Methylene Blue is utilized as a photosensitizer in Photodynamic Therapy (PDT). It exhibits a selective affinity for tumor tissues, allowing it to accumulate specifically in cancerous cells. When activated by light, Methylene Blue facilitates the destruction of these cancer cells.

Methylene Blue demonstrates antioxidant properties by effectively counteracting detrimental free radicals and diminishing cellular oxidative stress. Moreover, it has the potential to serve as a valuable tool for research and diagnostics by functioning as a staining agent that enables the identification and visualization of structures associated with oxidative stress. This includes mitochondria and reactive oxygen species (ROS), which are crucial in understanding various biological processes.

It is important to acknowledge that although Methylene Blue has demonstrated potential in these applications, additional research is currently being conducted to comprehensively comprehend its mechanisms of action and enhance its clinical utilization. The safe and effective use of Methylene Blue in medical and clinical settings relies heavily on factors such as proper dosage, administration, and consideration of individual patient characteristics.

Industrial and Scientific Applications of Methylene Blue

The unique properties and characteristics of Methylene Blue contribute to its wide range of industrial and scientific applications. Let's examine some of the prominent applications in these specific fields:

Methylene Blue is commonly used in a wide range of laboratory research applications. One potential application of this substance is its use as a staining agent, which allows for the visualization and differentiation of specific structures or cells when observed under a microscope. Histology commonly utilizes staining techniques to enhance the visibility of nuclei and other cellular components. Methylene Blue is commonly used in biochemical assays and molecular biology techniques for the purpose of identifying specific molecules or evaluating enzymatic activity.

The use of Methylene Blue as a dye or colorant is prevalent in the textile industry. The deep blue color of this dye is known for its ability to produce vibrant and long-lasting results when used to dye fabrics. The effectiveness of this product is notable when used on cotton, wool, and silk materials.

The dyeing process is a method where the fabric is submerged in a solution that contains Methylene Blue. This allows the dye molecules to attach themselves to the fibers of the fabric, resulting in the desired color.

Methylene Blue has been utilized in both photography and artistic practices. Black and white photography often utilizes contrast-enhancing agents to improve the sharpness and tonal range of the images. Moreover, the utilization of Methylene Blue extends to its application as a dye in alternative photographic techniques, including cyanotype or gum bichromate printing. In the realm of artistic practices, it is common to utilize it as a pigment or colorant in a variety of mediums.

Methylene Blue has been widely used in various environmental applications, with a particular focus on its effectiveness in water treatment processes. The antimicrobial properties and capacity to interact with organic molecules contribute to its efficacy in managing bacterial growth and eliminating contaminants.

Methylene Blue is commonly used in wastewater treatment processes due to its ability to effectively reduce bacterial loads and enhance water quality. The use of it is governed by specific regulations and considerations to ensure the treatment is safe and effective.

The redox indicator known as Methylene Blue is capable of undergoing reversible redox reactions by accepting or donating electrons. The property of this substance lends itself to practical applications in chemical analysis and titration processes. Specifically, it can be utilized to detect the existence of particular reducing or oxidizing agents. The color of Methylene Blue is dependent on its oxidation state, which enables the visual identification and measurement of redox reactions.

The concentration, purity, and specific formulations of Methylene Blue can vary in industrial applications, depending on the intended use. In industrial and scientific settings, it is crucial to prioritize safety and comply with regulations and guidelines when handling and disposing of Methylene Blue.

The broad range of applications for Methylene Blue in both industrial and scientific fields highlights its importance as a compound that extends beyond its medical uses. The unique properties of this substance contribute to its value in various industries, including staining, dyeing, analysis, and creative pursuits.

When it comes to safety, there are several important considerations and precautions that should be taken into account. These measures are crucial in order to prevent accidents, injuries, and potential

CHAPTER THREE

Safety Considerations and Precautions

To ensure safe and proper usage of Methylene Blue, it is crucial to adhere to safety considerations and precautions, thereby minimizing potential risks. The following safety guidelines are essential to consider:

It is important to wear the necessary personal protective equipment, such as gloves, safety goggles, and a lab coat or protective clothing, when handling Methylene Blue. The purpose of this is to provide protection for the skin, eyes, and clothing by preventing direct contact with the compound.

When dealing with Methylene Blue, it is important to exercise caution and take necessary precautions to prevent any unnecessary exposure or spills. It is recommended to store the item in a container that is tightly sealed to prevent any air or moisture from entering. It is important to keep the container in a cool and dry location, as exposure to heat or humidity can potentially degrade the item. Additionally, it is advisable to store the item away from direct sunlight, as prolonged exposure to sunlight can cause damage. It is also important to keep the item away from any substances that may react negatively with it, as this could potentially compromise its quality or safety. It is important to adhere to the manufacturer's instructions regarding storage conditions and shelf life.

It is important to ensure proper ventilation when working with Methylene Blue. This can be achieved by either working in a well-ventilated area or using fume hoods. The presence of proper ventilation is crucial in minimizing the risk of inhaling potentially hazardous vapors or dust particles.

It is important to note that the ingestion and inhalation of Methylene Blue should be avoided. It is advisable to refrain from eating, drinking, or smoking in areas where Methylene Blue is being utilized in order to minimize the risk of unintended ingestion. If someone accidentally ingests or inhales something, it is important to promptly seek medical attention.

It is important to avoid mixing Methylene Blue with substances or chemicals that are incompatible, as this can result in hazardous reactions. It is important to adhere to appropriate chemical segregation practices in order to avoid any unintended mixing.

Proper disposal of Methylene Blue and any materials contaminated with it should be carried out in compliance with local regulations and guidelines for waste disposal. It is advisable to seek guidance from local authorities or waste management facilities regarding appropriate methods for disposing of waste.

It is possible for certain individuals to experience allergic reactions or sensitivities to Methylene Blue. Individuals who have a confirmed sensitivity or allergy to dyes or related compounds should take necessary precautions or explore alternative options. If you experience any negative reactions, stop using the product and consult a medical professional.

First Aid: When there is skin contact, it is important to promptly cleanse the affected area by washing it with soap and water. In the event of eye contact with Methylene Blue, it is recommended to rinse the eyes with water for several minutes, ensuring that the eyelids are kept open. In the event that irritation continues, it is advisable to consult with a medical professional. If someone accidentally ingests or inhales something, it is important to promptly seek medical help.

It is crucial to acknowledge that the aforementioned guidelines pertain to general safety considerations. However, it is important to recognize that specific precautions may differ based on factors such as the concentration, form, and intended use of Methylene Blue. It is important to consistently consult the safety data sheet (SDS) provided by the manufacturer in order to access comprehensive safety information and instructions.

Adhering to safety considerations and precautions is crucial for maintaining the safe handling, storage, and use of Methylene Blue. This approach helps to minimize potential risks and create a secure working environment.

CHAPTER FOUR

Emerging Research and Future Perspectives

Ongoing research on Methylene Blue is revealing additional knowledge and exploring various potential uses for this adaptable compound. The following areas of study and future perspectives for Methylene Blue are worth considering:

Methylene Blue has demonstrated potential in studies investigating neurodegenerative diseases, including Alzheimer's and Parkinson's. According to studies, there is evidence to suggest that it could have potential benefits in mitigating oxidative stress, reducing neuroinflammation, and improving mitochondrial function. These effects may have the potential to slow down the progression of diseases or provide relief from symptoms. Ongoing research is focused on investigating the neuroprotective effects and therapeutic potential of this substance in these conditions.

Methylene Blue is currently under investigation for its potential role as an adjunct in cancer therapies. Studies have indicated that Methylene Blue, apart from its role as a photosensitizer in photodynamic therapy, may possess direct anticancer properties. These properties include the ability to impede the growth of cancer cells and facilitate apoptosis. The use of this treatment is being investigated by researchers in combination with other therapeutic agents to improve treatment outcomes.

Antimicrobial resistance has become a significant concern, leading to an increased focus on exploring alternative antimicrobial agents. Methylene Blue has been found to possess antimicrobial properties that are effective against a wide range of bacteria and fungi. Future research could potentially prioritize the investigation of the effectiveness of this treatment against drug-resistant strains and the development of novel approaches to address the issue of antimicrobial resistance.

According to certain studies, there is evidence to suggest that Methylene Blue might have potential benefits in terms of aiding wound healing and tissue regeneration. The potential of this subject to stimulate angiogenesis (the process of forming new blood vessels) and improve wound healing has been thoroughly examined. Future research could focus on investigating and improving the effectiveness of Methylene Blue formulations and delivery methods in order to enhance therapeutic outcomes in the context of wound healing applications.

Photodynamic antiviral therapy has emerged as a promising approach for the treatment of viral infections in recent years. The potential of Methylene

Blue as a photosensitizer for photodynamic antiviral therapy is being investigated by researchers. This therapy utilizes light activation to deactivate viruses. The field of study mentioned shows potential in addressing viral infections that are challenging to manage using traditional antiviral medications.

The redox properties of Methylene Blue make it a desirable option for energy storage and conversion applications. The use of this material is being studied by researchers in redox flow batteries and as a catalyst in electrochemical systems for energy storage and conversion, such as fuel cells and supercapacitors. The objective of these studies is to utilize the distinctive characteristics of this subject in order to develop energy technologies that are both more sustainable and efficient.

As research advances in these areas, it is possible that Methylene Blue will continue to exhibit its potential in diverse fields. Ongoing studies and future perspectives indicate potential for the expansion of applications and the discovery of new therapeutic and technological advancements.

Methylene Blue exhibits versatility as a compound, displaying a diverse array of applications and potential advantages. The unique properties of this substance, such as its ability to stain, its redox properties, and its antimicrobial effects, contribute to its value in diverse fields such as medicine, research, and industry.

Methylene Blue is commonly used as a diagnostic dye in the medical and clinical field. It helps with the visualization and differentiation of tissues and biological specimens. Additionally, it is utilized in the medical management of methemoglobinemia, a medical condition characterized by a decrease in the blood's ability to carry oxygen. In addition, there is ongoing research that indicates potential neuroprotective effects of this substance. Additionally, it is being studied for its potential use in photodynamic therapy for specific types of cancers.

Methylene Blue is commonly utilized in the industrial sector, specifically in the textile industry, for its dyeing and coloring properties. Additionally, it is utilized in the fields of photography and artistic practices, providing benefits such as contrast enhancement and alternative printing methods. Moreover, the antimicrobial properties of the substance render it valuable in various water treatment and environmental applications.

It is essential to have a thorough understanding of the safety considerations and precautions related to Methylene Blue in order to handle and use it correctly. Ensuring compliance with guidelines pertaining to personal protective equipment, storage, disposal, and chemical incompatibilities is crucial for maintaining a safe working environment.

Ongoing research is currently investigating the potential applications of Methylene Blue in various areas, including neurodegenerative diseases, anticancer therapies, antimicrobial resistance, wound healing, and energy storage. These potential uses present exciting possibilities for the future of Methylene Blue. Further benefits and advancements in the field may be unlocked through continued investigations into the mechanisms of action and optimization of clinical applications.

The versatility of Methylene Blue, along with its established applications and ongoing research, underscores its importance across different domains. The compound's distinct characteristics and wide range of applications make it an intriguing subject for scientists, medical professionals, researchers, and industries. This opens up possibilities for future advancements and breakthroughs.

The medical applications and notable potential of methylene blue encompass a wide range of uses, including but not limited to:

Malaria is a potentially life-threatening disease caused by parasites that are transmitted to humans through the It has been observed that methylene blue exhibits efficacy in the treatment of malaria.

Impairment of cognitive function resulting in the inability to recall or retain information. In addition to its potential benefits in dementia, methylene blue has been found to possess antioxidant properties that may assist in mitigating age-related damage that accrues gradually.

Lyme disease: The study focused on pharmaceutical interventions targeting the eradication of the causative bacteria responsible for Lyme disease. In the laboratory setting, it was observed that methylene blue demonstrated efficacy in eradicating antibiotic-resistant bacteria.

Cancer detection has been employed for the identification of gastrointestinal cancers, overactive parathyroid glands, and cancerous growths within lymph nodes.

Alzheimer's disease: Researchers are currently investigating the potential of methylene to mitigate memory decline in individuals diagnosed with Alzheimer's dementia.

END